Very Effective Ways to Lose Weight Without Exercise

Facts, Methods, The Best Weight Loss Diets and Top 7 The Best Fat Burning Recipes

Table of Contents

Introduction 1

13 Facts and Researches 5

Advantages of Losing Weigh 14

Methods in Losing Weight Without Exercise 17

Top 7: The Best Weight-Loss Diets Ever...............20

    Green Smoothies 21

    Ingredients for Weight Loss...................... 21

    Ingredients to Avoid 23

    Green Smoothie Recipes 24

Effective Eating Habits 30

    Day 1: Low-Sugar Fruit Day 32

    Day 2: Vegetable Diet 33

    Day 3: Fruits and Vegetables 35

    Day 4: Banana's Best............................. 37

    Day 5: Tomato Mania 39

    Day 6: Rice, Vegetable, and Soup............... 41

    Day 7: Rice, Soup and Juice Diet................ 42

Top 7 Life Hacks in Losing Weight Without
Exercise 44

Conclusion...47

Introduction

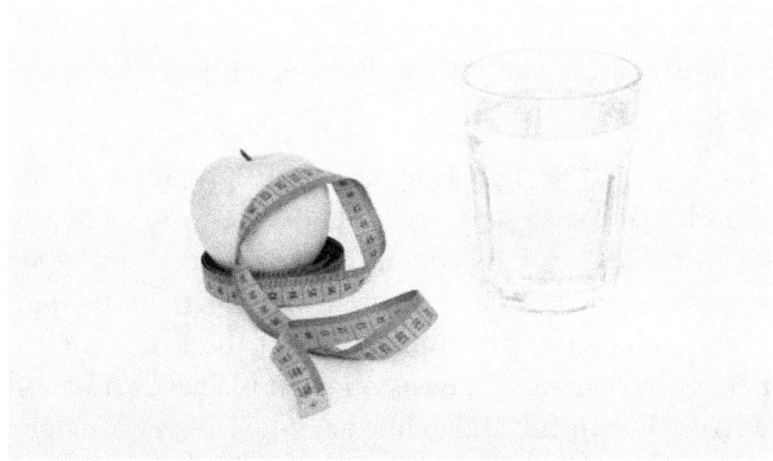

Dr. Steve Maraboli once said, "The healthy life: It is not just about losing the weight; it is about losing the lifestyle and mindset that you got there." Losing weight does not happen overnight, and it is far from being an easy process. Losing weight means persistence, determination, and self-control. So, unless you want to stay overweight or obese, ask yourself? Am I willing to change for my own future? Am I willing to do everything in my power to free myself from negative thinking and unhealthy habits? If you are, you have come to the right place.

Weight loss in the medical context, refers to the reduction of the body's total mass due to loss of fluid, body fat, adipose tissues, or lean mass such as bone mineral deposits, muscles, tendons, and other connective tissues. It is further defined by MedicineNet.com as the decrease in body weight from voluntary or involuntary circumstances. Voluntary circumstances include exercise and diet. However, involuntary circumstances include being sick or having a disease such as cancer, typhoid, malabsorption and other illnesses as a way to lose weight.

According to Weight Concern (2017), there are many possible reasons why an individual chooses to lose weight. The first reason is being fit and sexy. The society nowadays have created their own status quo. Due to the widespread influence of the social media, people have created a basis on what is sexy or not; and what is beautiful and what is not. The reason why other people want to lose weight is because they want to feel beautiful and they want to feel accepted in the society. They believe that being sexy and slim is "in" and attractive in their environment. Other people want to get rid of the different names people call them. They want to get noticed. They want appreciation. And they want to fit in.

More to the point, other people want to stay healthy and sexy because they want to fit into their old clothes. Some, they want to put on sexy and revealing attires, even to wear bikinis without being ashamed of doing so. Others, they want to impress and attract other people to them. But whatever their motives are, losing weight is not only good for the external appearance of the body, it also helps the body to function effectively and efficiently on the inside.

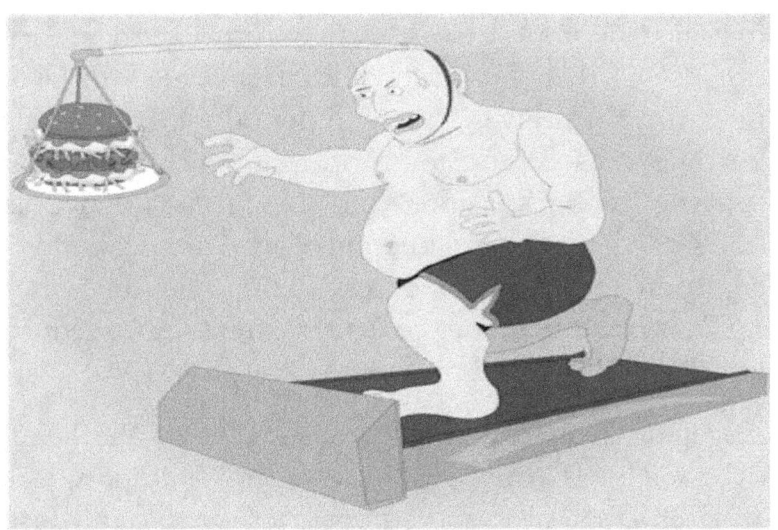

Obesity and being overweight can cause detrimental conditions for the body. It can cause an individual to be more prone to diabetes, heart failures, kidney failures, and other diseases. This is also one of the top reasons why losing weight is essential. They want to build and maintain a healthy diet to finally get rid of their medications. Other people also want to lose weight because they want to prevent being ill before it is too late. One of its advantages includes saving money from purchasing various medicines, visiting doctors, and buying unhealthy food. People who think about losing weight this way believe that health is indeed wealth. Not only does losing weight save you money but also help you aid and prevent medical conditions.

In this busy world where we live in, there is a very fine line between the time for work and time for oneself. People nowadays work two to three shifts in a day just to make a living for themselves and their family. And because of their busy schedule, they neglect to have time for themselves. Often times, these individuals become stressed and tend to engage in binge-eating activities or stress eating. Binge-eating is defined as one's tendency to eat uncontrollably due to various environmental factors. Stress eating, on the other hand, is one's tendency to eat the stress out to reduce internal and external pressure.

Engaging in these activities causes obesity and being overweight. If you already are in this condition, it is apparent that you take control of yourself and lose some weight. Time management is no longer an issue, for there are already different ways on how to lose weight without exercise. You do not have to spare time and money to go to the gym or to jog every morning. You no longer have to invest on accessories and machines to help you lose weight at home. This is due to the fact that life innovations nowadays have found out various ways and methods to lose weight effectively without exercise. So, if you are the kind of person who would rather stay on the couch all day, or if you are the kind of person who just wants to work a lot but wants to lose weight, then you have purchased the right book. For in the following chapters, you will realize that losing weight will no longer be a problem as long as you stay committed, persistent and determined to become the person you ought to be.

13 Facts and Researches

To some people, losing weight is just that – coming out being slimmer and leaner for losing fat. But just like other concepts and topics, losing weight also has different myths and different facts attached to it. According to one article from the Reader's Digest written by Joanne Chen (2017), there are thirteen things that people did not know about weight loss.

The first fact is that losing weight is really genetic. Some people find it easier to lose weight than others because of their genetic predisposition. If they carry a gene which enables them to lose fat by small and simple means, then it could manifest in their body's physiology and it could also throughout the family's lineage. However, there are people who tend to carry a gene which enables them to lose fat more slowly than others. Some of these people struggle so much to lose weight yet they are still granted minimum improvement. To some, this seems unfair. But that's the reality of life. If losing weight is not easy for you, then you have to be extra tenacious in the process. You have to rethink your attitudes in order to maximize its effects.

The second fact is that some people have more fat cells than others. People who have more tend to find losing weight even more difficult than others. Fat cells emerge during childhood, especially for girls because most of them are more reserved, unlike boys who are known to be more active. People who have more fat cells have to go through a much harder and longer process to get rid of their fat cells for good.

The third study is about metabolism. Did you know that you can change your own metabolism? According to Dr. KirsiPietilainen from Helsinki University Central Hospital, the more fat you gain, the harder it is to lose it. He conducted a study on two identical twins in which the other is fat the other is slim. They soon observed that the overweight twin has a slower metabolism than the slim one. This proves that excess fat can really influence one's metabolism. However, when one slowly reduces his amount of body fat, this will also entail a faster metabolism which will aid in a faster road to being physically fit and sexy.

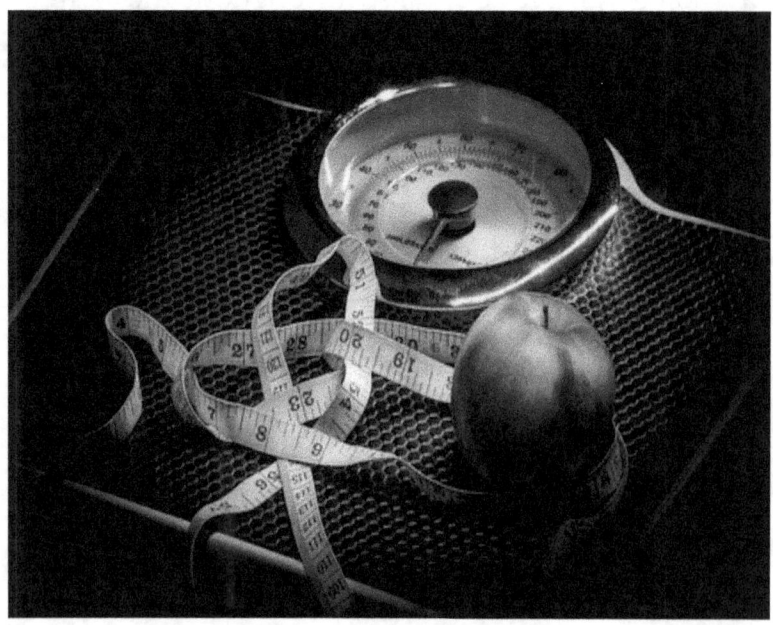

Furthermore, researchers have proven that stress can really make someone stout. According to studies, stress hormones incline up fat storage. This is the main reason why people who are stressed tend to eat more than they used to because they want to give themselves the satisfaction of relief. Other people consider stress-eating as their last resort when they are being pressured, anxious or apprehended in their jobs or in their various daily activities. If you are one of the individuals who stress eat so much, try to find a different outlet for your stress such as playing video games, writing or drawing, doing house chores – anything to prevent you from having the food-in-the-mouth syndrome which makes you eat a lot in stressful situations.

Another must-known fact is that your mother's pregnancy causes a huge effect on your body mass. Remember the concept which states that pregnant women who smoke and drink alcohol can cause damage to their offspring at birth? This is the same case for body fat. How your mom eats during pregnancy affect the amount of fat in your body. So, if your mother was eating a lot of sugary, fatty and unhealthy foods while she was pregnant with you, it will no longer be a surprise if you are born stout. If the body fats persist inside you until your adolescence, it will be harder for you to lose more weight. This is the reason why mothers should ensure and implement proper diet for their children at a young age to help them achieve and maintain a normal weight while they are still young. Prior to that, they are also recommended to eat well for their unborn baby to prevent the adverse effects that an unhealthy diet can provide.

Sleep is also one of the main factors that affect weight. According to Louis Aronne, MD, people should sleep for seven to eight hours. People who sleep less tend to grow fat because sleep deprivation inhibits hormonal balance. Apart from that, it triggers the decrease in Leptin (the hormone that helps you feel full) and the increase in Ghrelin (the hormone that makes you feel hungry). Because of this imbalance, you will feel that you are hungry even when you are not. This causes overeating. Therefore, the chance of gaining fat is at its peak.

Another study in the New England Journal indicates that weight gain and weight loss can be contagious. If you are with people who tend to eat a lot, then you are more likely to join them. However, if you are with a crowd who is more health conscious, then this might motivate you to lose weight and maintain a good body shape. One theory that can explain this phenomenon is the Social Learning Theory by Albert Bandura. This states that an individual learns from what he sees, hears or observes. The environment can influence an individual's actions and attitudes due to learning. And as motivated people who want to lose weight, you can start by being with people who can motivate you do so. Stay with people who are determined to be in shape and to be physically fit. In no time, you will be one of them too.

Furthermore, according to Dr. Dhurandhar from Pennington, viral infections seem to increase the number of fat cells in the body as well as its content. One of the most famous virus that can cause obesity is Adenovirus which is responsible for a host of ills from the upper respiratory tract to the gastrointestinal tubes. It has been found that cells inflicted with a strain of virus can fatten them all up. This will cause the expansion of body fat. All the more reason to stay in shape! You would not want to be prone to several illnesses, wouldn't you?

Did you know that food can be as addictive as alcohol and drugs? Researchers from Brookhaven National Laboratory in Upton, New York found that food can stimulate the production of dopamine – the hormone linked to motivation and pleasure. It has been studied that obese people have fewer dopamine receptors, which makes them eat more food to maintain their homeostasis and produce supplemental dopamine in their body. It is also observed that people who are overweight and obese tend to have lower self-confidence and self-esteem. This might also be the result of having a lower amount of dopamine in the bloodstream. The reason why they eat it out is to increase their amount of sugar in their body and produce dopamine to make them feel more alive and happy.

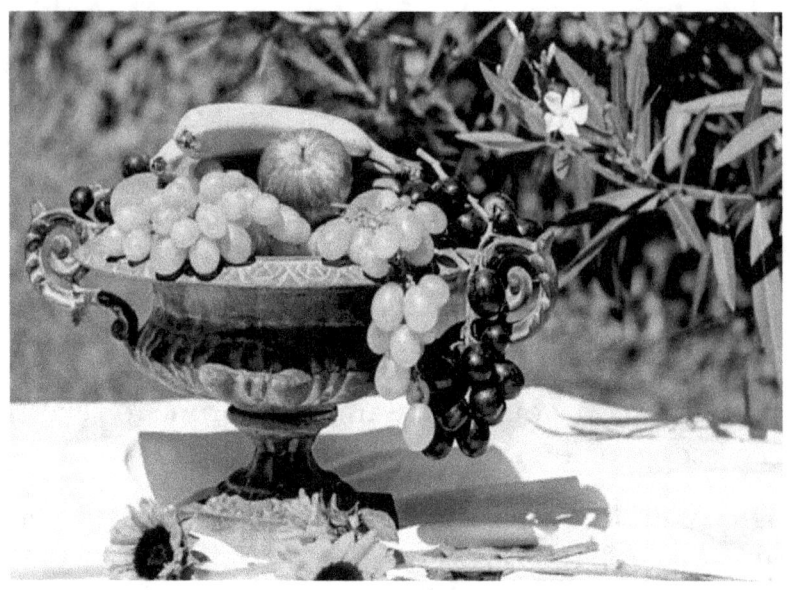

Further researches also added that having ear infections can make you stouter. The reason behind is that these types of infections can affect the taste buds of an individual. When one's taste buds are impaired, they tend to taste everything as bland. Therefore, they like to increase the sweetness of the food that they eat which means adding sugar and other unhealthy condiments to their diet. If you too are having this condition, then you should find healthier food substitutes like fruits, olive oil, and butter instead of junk food and sweets. This might even help you lose weight more.

Moreover, Zane Andrews from Monash University stated that free radicals do not only make you look older but also make you stouter. These oxidizing molecules damage the cells that tell us that we are already full. This makes us become even more hungry and engage in unhealthy eating habits. It has also been found that the emergence of free radicals is at its peak when people eat a lot of candy bars, chips, and other carbohydrates. So, instead of gorging onto these destructive foods, why not try something better such as fruits and vegetables? These will not only make you look glowing on the outside, but it can also help you lose weight.

Gurus from all over the world have coined four basic rules to a healthy eating habit. The first one is to consume carbs in the form of whole grains and fiber such as oats, brown rice, rye, etc. These will aid for a better digestion and a better body structure. Eating whole grains and fiber-rich food provide good carbs, and produces a low-calorie intake. The second rule is to avoid trans-fat and saturated fats. Trans fat raises your low-density lipoprotein or bad cholesterol which is detrimental to your health. Most trans-fat are in the form of hydrogenated oil which is found in baked goods, snacks, fried food, refrigerator dough, creamer and margarine. Saturated fats however increase blood cholesterol which is responsible for atherosclerosis, which is the blockage of the veins or arteries due to cholesterol and fat build-up. Common foods with saturated fats include fatty beef, lamb, pork, poultry with skin, lard and cream, butter and cheese.

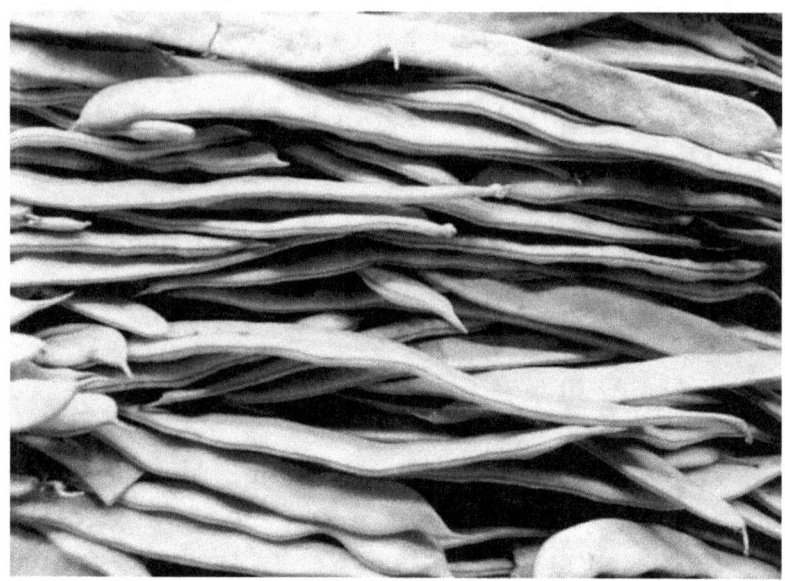

The third rule is to eat lean protein such as dairy, beans, eggs, soy foods, nuts and seeds. This aid to keep hunger stable and regular which provides control to the body's production of leptin and ghrelin. Keeping the hunger at bay in between meals will prevent temptations of over eating and binge eating which results to a good weight maintenance and a good form of weight loss. And the last rule is to eat lots of fruits and vegetables. These foods are proven to aid in digestion. These also help increase the number of vitamins and minerals in the body. It can help you lose weight and at the same time assist you in keeping the essential nutrients within.

And the last fact states that an individual can be fat, yet fit. If you are stout, it does not mean that you are unhealthy. Conversely, if you are lean and slim, it does not mean that you are healthy. According to a study published in the Archives of Internal Medicine, that among 5440 individuals, 51% of the overweight and almost 32% of the obese had normal cholesterol, blood sugar, blood pressure and other measures of good health. They also found that 23.5% of slim adults were metabolically abnormal, making them more vulnerable to heart disease and other illnesses. Being physically fit is indeed based on someone's lifestyle, not someone's weight. Be careful not to overwork yourself in trying to be slim. There might be a time when you might have lost your weight, but you also lost your good health.

Advantages of Losing Weigh

For some people, they think that losing weight is just a means of fitting into smaller jeans and shirts. Others think that it is just essential for attracting men and women. Well according to researchers, there are many surprising benefits of weight loss. Gagnon (2017) from Men's Fitness, one of the best advantages of weight loss is better sleep and better hormonal balance. Studies show that losing 5% of body weight can help people sleep better and longer through the night. It also prevents one from sleep apnea and snoring. Weight loss is also good for the production of an essential hormone called the thyroxine secreted by the thyroid glands. It is responsible for the body's metabolism which is the process of breaking down of food and the absorption of essential nutrients.

Furthermore, studies also prove that losing weight can decrease the prevalence of joint pain. The skeletal frame and joints carry the body mass of your body from your excess fats. Once you lose these your bones, tendons, and ligaments no longer have to carry the same amount of weight and are therefore relieved of strenuous pressure. The healthier food intake which results in weight loss also contribute to a clearer, and brighter skin. Foods like fruits and vegetables help avoid acne and clogged pores, making the skin, supple and radiant on the outside.

Losing weight also entails stress relief because it enables you to sleep tight, and eat a balanced diet.

With this lifestyle, the body will be more resilient to pressure, anxiety, and apprehension which are the main causes of stress. It is also very helpful in preventing various illnesses and diseases such as colds, cough, cancer, diabetes, and heart failure. Weight loss is also proven to help improve memory. It helps the brain process faster, sharper and more alert due to the production of dopamine and endorphin in the body.

The practical advantages of weight loss include saving money, fitting into old and new clothes, and gaining more friends. First of all, you will be able to save money from buying expensive junk foods. Instead, you will only be inclined to purchase fruits, vegetables and other healthy foods which are cheaper in the marketplace. You will also spare yourself from spending lots of money for various medicines and check-ups. Losing weight also means being more fashionable because you can gain the confidence wear whatever you like whenever you want it. You will never feel as conscious as before because you already have the body you aspire. And lastly, you can gain more friends from losing weight not only because of the change of appearance but also the change in mood. Losing weight increases the production of the happy hormone, endorphin, which will give you the chance to let people be with you and have fun.

There are literally lots of advantages of losing weight. Researchers even believe that it is good for an individual's longevity. Whatever your reasons are for losing weight, be sure to stick with it and remember all of these wonderful advantages. This might provide additional motivation to your journey towards a slim, lean and healthy body. Get rid of your negativities. And always keep in mind to make healthy living a habit.

Methods in Losing Weight Without Exercise

As stated before, people nowadays are on a tight schedule. Some people no longer have enough time for themselves much less a gym or a jog. This book emphasizes very effective ways to lose weight without exercise. So, no matter where you go or what you do, you can make sure that you are doing something productive towards the improvement of your body.

Another very effective method in pushing yourself away from unhealthy foods is to keep them out of sight. Putting these junk foods where you can see them will cause temptation, and therefore enticing you to eat more. Or better yet, do not purchase unhealthy foods. It is better if you place healthy foods where you can see them. In this manner, you can control yourself and push yourself to resort back to eating healthier foods.

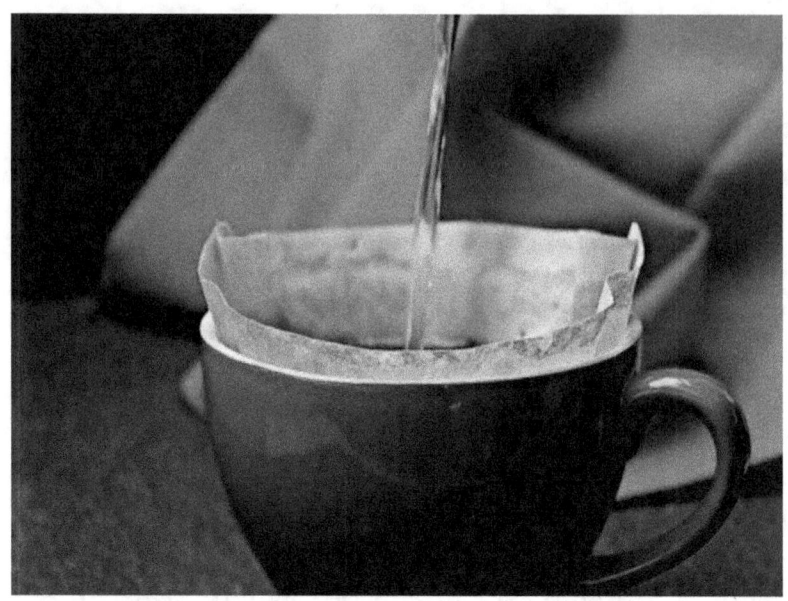

Furthermore, viscous fiber is also an effective means to lose weight. Like proteins, they also help someone feel full and therefore, eat less. Viscous fiber forms a gel-like texture when it takes contact with water which increases the amount of time to absorb nutrients in the stomach. This also helps slow down the emptying of the stomach to feel satiated in a longer period of time. Examples of viscous fiber include beans, oat cereals, Brussel sprouts, asparagus, oranges and flax seeds.

Drinking water is also one of the best ways to lose weight because it helps flush out the excess toxins in the body. Studies show that drinking half a liter of water (17 oz) thirty minutes before meals can reduce hunger, decreasing the amount of calorie intake. People who drank water before meals lost 44% more weight in 12 weeks compared to others who did not.

The next eating habit is to serve yourself smaller portions to decrease the amount of food intake. Researchers show that doubling the size of a dinner starter increases the calorie intake by 30%. Larger portion sizes are linked to being obese and overweight. This is the reason why everyone is encouraged to serve themselves smaller portions for control and weight loss.

Pay attention to what you eat. Often times, when people are watching TV or playing videogames while eating, they tend to feel the urge to eat more. This will then cause an increased calorie intake. Studies showed that people who are distracted during a meal ate 10% more than usual in that one sitting. It has also been proven that people who are distracted during meals eat 25% more calories at later meals than those who are not distracted.

You should sleep well and avoid stress. Not having enough sleep and being stressed causes the body to have hormonal imbalance causing an elevation to your hunger and cravings for unhealthy food. Eliminate your consumption of various sugar-filled drinks. These consists of massive levels of calories due to the many ingredients and unhealthy condiments present. Sugary drinks are linked to increased weight gain and many diseases. So, instead of drinking soda, try water, coffee, and tea instead.

Top 7: The Best Weight-Loss Diets Ever

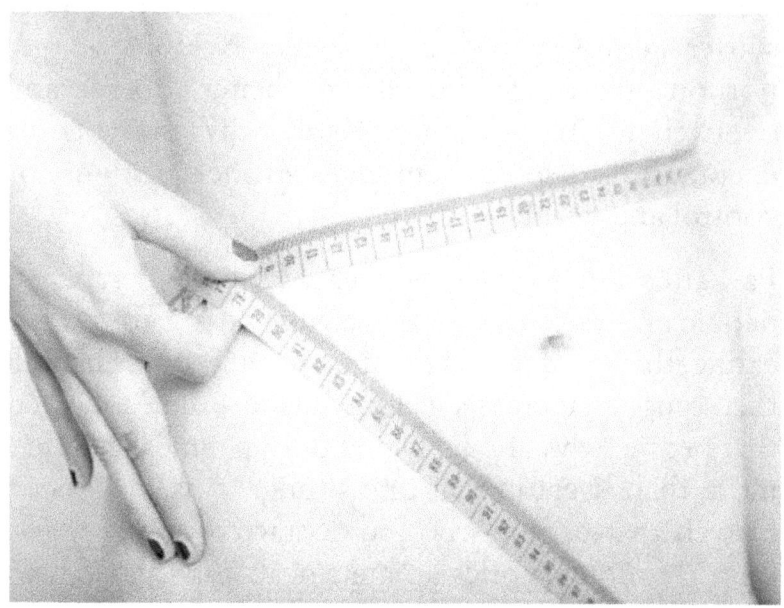

In this chapter, you will see the top seven weight loss diet plan you can use to lose weight within seven days (Harris, 2017). These recipes will not only help you become healthier but also make you slimmer and leaner without exercise. The nutritional content of these recipes is enough to sustain your strength and energy in a day, and at the same time get rid of the excess fats you want to trim. But before you start, let me be the first one to tell you that it is not going to be easy. Especially when you are used to other forms of diet. For this process to take effect, and for you to gain promising results, you have to really commit. This diet plan with recipes are already proven to trim your fats and help you achieve your desired weight.

All you need to do is persist and persevere until day seven, and lose ten pounds instantly.

Green Smoothies

When people think about smoothies, they only often think of it as a means to quench thirst or to ease the body from warm temperatures. What they do not know is green smoothies are actually one of the best ways of losing weight because you, yourself control the ingredients. Green smoothies are filled with low-calorie, nutrient-filled ingredients which are capable of sustaining a healthy body.

According to Camody (2017), the reason why smoothies are the best recipes for weight loss is that they have a good balance of protein, carbohydrates, healthy fats, vitamins and nutrients. You can also add powerhouse ingredients to get you pumped up without increasing the amount of calorie intake. In that way, you can boost your metabolic rate and energy.

The Healthy Smoothie Headquarters included the different ingredients for a smoothie that we should add and avoid for weight loss:

Ingredients for Weight Loss

1. Avocado – This fruit supply healthy fat which helps you feel satiated in between meals. This will aid to avoid temptation in eating until your next meal hours.

2. Berries – These do not only add flavor to the smoothie but also provide fiber and antioxidants for the body to function more effectively.

3. Cayenne Pepper – Aside from adding spice to the smoothie, it also helps you boost your weight loss capability. It reduces the consumption of fat and carbohydrates when taken during breakfast because it helps you control your appetite.

4. Chia Seeds – These tiny seeds are rich in fiber and protein that aid in digestion. It is also filled with nutrients such as calcium, antioxidants, and omega-3 fatty acids.

5. Cinnamon – This is one of the famous ingredients of smoothies not because of the taste but also of its innate capability to regulate blood sugar levels that can be stored as fats.

6. Coconut Oil – The fats that consist from coconut are not stored as fat but rather converted to energy. Furthermore, it does not only promote weight loss but also optimal health.

7. Yogurt – These are high in protein that can fill you up and keep you full in a long period of time.

8. Leafy Greens – Kale, spinach, dandelion, and lettuce are some of the greens that are filled

with phytonutrients, fiber and are low in calories.

9. Fruits – These are one of the most essential ingredients of smoothies because they promote healthy digestion. They also provide a wide variety of minerals and nutrients without increasing the number of calories.

10. Tea – Tea is known to be one of the most detoxifying ingredient of smoothies. It helps clean out the excess fat and nutrients from the body. It is also essential in promoting a good digestion and bowel movement.

Ingredients to Avoid

1. Canned fruits and vegetables – These are filled with preservatives and sweeteners which increases the number of calories. They also have lost a significant amount of nutritional value due to their processing and packing.

2. Dairy – These are chock full of calories. However, there can be exceptions such as Greek yogurt and raw milk which are high in protein but low in sugar.

3. Fruit juice –High in sugar and calories but low in nutritional value. Increasing the amount of fruit juice intake will also increase your bad calorie intake.

4. Sweeteners – Sugar can increase our calorie intake. If you like your smoothie to be sweet,

use stevia. It is a natural, low-calorie sweetener that you can use.

5. Too much sweet fruit – You should also take into consideration the sweetness of the fruit you put on your smoothie. Having too much sweet fruits will cause sugar and digestive problems. Better stick to banana, mango, pineapple and other fruits to better promote weight loss.

Green Smoothie Recipes

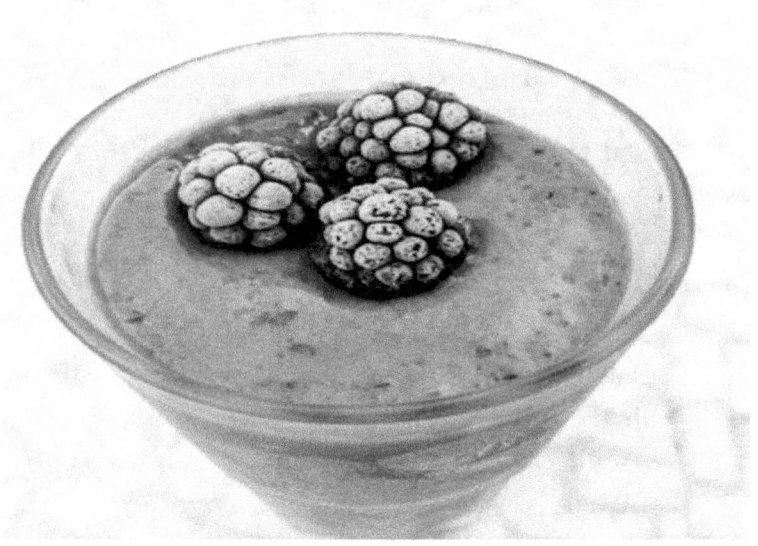

According to Lose Weight by Eating (2017), the process of drinking smoothie for weight loss means replacing 1 or 2 meals a day with smoothie recipe. In this way, you can easily lose weight in as fast as 5-10 pounds in 3 days. Weight loss smoothies or green smoothies are responsible for detoxification that enable you to get rid of toxins, excess fats and nutrients. With a good smoothie blender, you are ready to start with one of the most delicious forms of losing weight.

Ryan's Ideal Weight Loss Smoothie:

- 1 cup water
- 1/2 medium avocado
- 1/2 cup fresh or frozen blueberries
- 1 tablespoon chia seeds or chia seed gel
- 1/2 tablespoon coconut oil (increase to 1 tablespoon over the course of a week)
- 1/4 teaspoon cinnamon
- 1/2 tablespoon honey (optionally use stevia or maple syrup or 1/2 banana to sweeten)

Mango Avocado Green Tea Smoothie

- 1 cup green tea
- 1 cup fresh or frozen mango chunks
- 1/2 medium avocado
- 1 cup spinach
- 1/2 tablespoon coconut oil
- A dash of sea salt

- A little honey, maple syrup, or stevia to sweeten (optional, mango provides enough sweet for me

Blueberry Greek Yogurt Smoothie

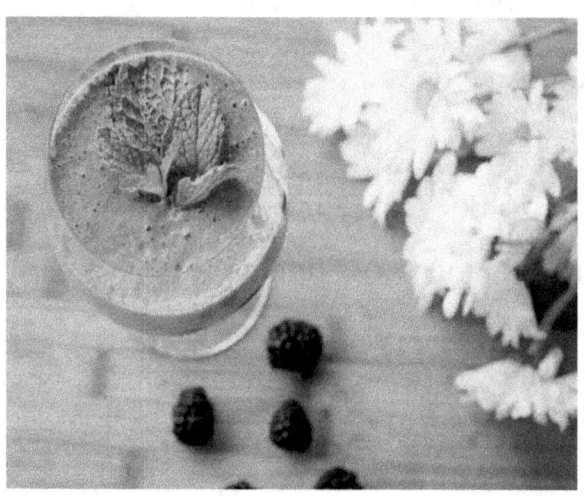

- 1/2 cup water

- 1/2 cup fresh or frozen blueberries

- 3/4 cup of plain, Greek yogurt (preferably full-fat)

- 1 tablespoon chia seeds or chia seed gel

- 1/4 teaspoon cinnamon

- 1/2 tablespoon honey (optionally use stevia or maple syrup or 1/2 banana to sweeten)

Berry Banana Smoothie

- 1 cup water

- 1 cup fresh or frozen mixed berries

- 1/2 fresh or frozen banana

- 1 cup spinach

- 1 tablespoon coconut oil

- 1/4 teaspoon cayenne pepper

- 1 tablespoon gelatin (optional, for protein)

Green Protein Detox Smoothie

- ½ cup unsweetened almond milk

- 1 tablespoon almond butter

- 1 banana

- 2 cups mixed greens (I like kale, chard and spinach)

Glowing Green Detox Smoothie

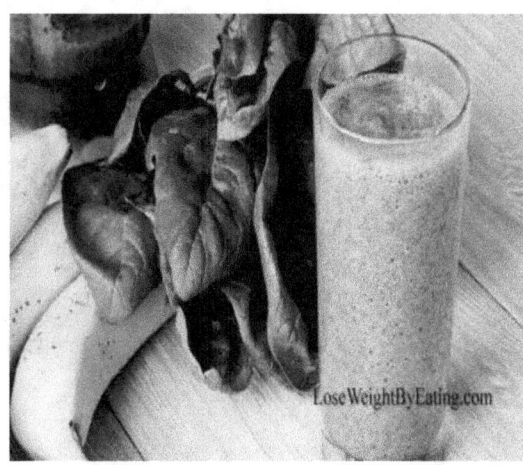

- 1 kiwi
- 1 banana
- ¼ cup pineapple
- 2 celery stalks
- 2 cups spinach
- 1 cup water

Apple Berry Detox Smoothie

- 1 cup mixed berries (like raspberries, strawberries, and blueberries)
- 1 large apple
- 2 cups spinach
- 1 cup water (or unsweetened almond milk)

Pineapple Banana Detox Smoothie

- 1 cup pineapple
- 1 banana
- 1 apple
- 2 cups spinach
- 1 cup water

Kale and Apple Green Detox Smoothie

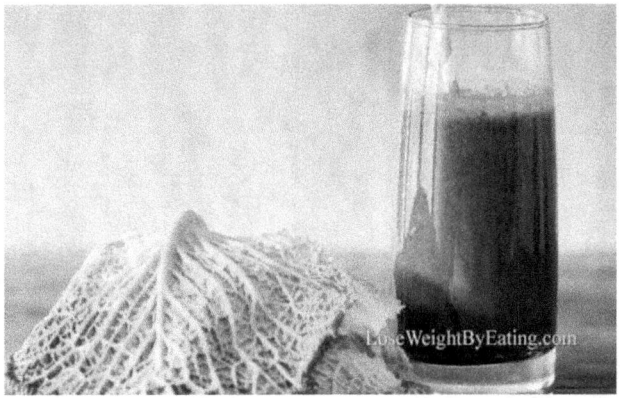

- ⅔ cup almond milk (unsweetened)
- ¾ cup ice
- 1 ½ cups kale (chopped)
- 1 stalk celery (chopped)
- ½ red or green apple (cored and chopped)
- 1 tbsp ground flax seed
- 1 teaspoon honey (optional)

Kale Strawberry Banana Detox Smoothie

- 1 banana
- 1 cup yogurt (plain)
- 1 cup strawberries (fresh or frozen)
- 1 cup Kale (chopped)
- 1 cup ice

Effective Eating Habits

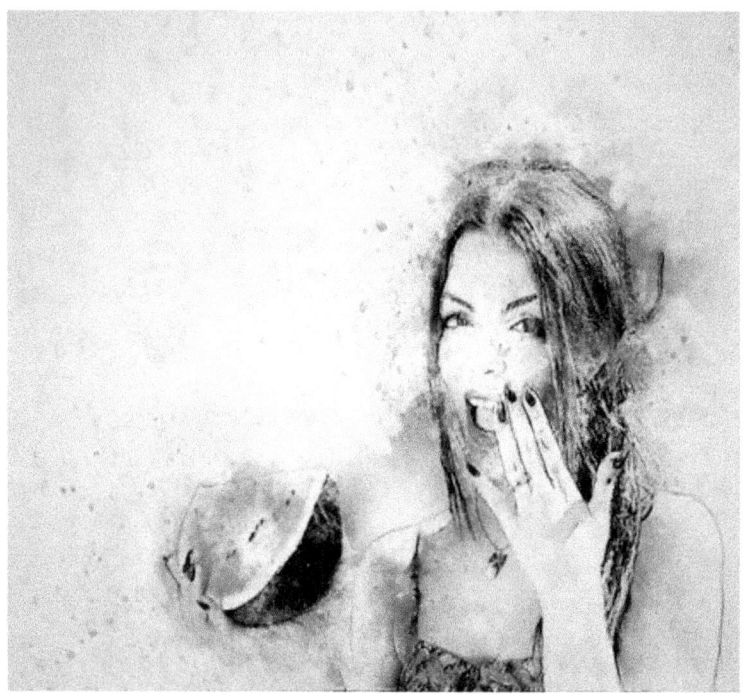

Aside from green smoothies, there are also various eating habits that you can incorporate with your diet. These eating habits are essential in one's journey to weight loss because it entails discipline and persistence. These habits also constitute ways on how you can improve your weight loss strategies. Simple as these actions are, they are still very effective especially when they are executed in a regular and healthy manner. These eating habits will help you trim down the absorption of fats in the body which will enable a better metabolism on the road to losing weight.

According to Palsdottir (2016) from Authority Nutrition, there are different proven ways to lose weight without diet or exercise. The first one is to chew thoroughly and slowly. Chewing your food better will decrease food intake because it gives the feeling of fullness and satiation. 23 observational studies prove that people who eat faster are more likely to gain weight than those who eat slowly.

Using smaller plates for unhealthy foods such as sweets and food with preservatives is also a good way to control your calorie intake. It will also motivate you to eat less unhealthy food and focus more on healthy foods such as fruits and vegetables. In using smaller plates for unhealthy foods, it will seem that you are already eating more than you should. This will cause you to eat less.

Researchers also added that protein constitutes a powerful effect on one's appetite. It can intensify the feeling of satiation, reduce hunger and help consume fewer calories. According to a study, increasing the amount of protein from 15% to 30%causes fewer calorie intake and helps lose around 11 pounds to 12 pounds in one week without exercise. Protein-rich foods include salmon, lean beef and chicken breasts, tuna and cottage cheese.

Day 1: Low-Sugar Fruit Day

By the end of the day, be sure that you've eaten at least four apples, four oranges, one slice of watermelon and two pomegranates. The allowed beverages for seven days include at least 10 glasses of water, green tea, and coffee.

Fruits are keys to a healthy digestion. They are effective detoxifiers and helps well in weight loss. Did you know that Grapefruit is the best weigh loss fruit? It is low in sugar content and is filled with fiber. It may taste acidic, but it's one risk you should take on the road to losing weight. Apples, when combined with other fruits are great ways to lose weight. They contain pectin which aids in the digestive system's bowel movement. They also contain phosphorous and potassium to help flush out toxins and excess fats from the body.

For a weight loss drink you can add to your diet for seven days, Mix two tablespoons of honey into a glass of warm water. Add three tablespoons of freshly squeezed lemon juice. Mix well and drink before breakfast every day this week.

Day 2: Vegetable Diet

This day's recipe focuses on vegetables. It is up to you if you'd like them raw plain, boiled or salted. But you should avoid cream, butter, milk and oil. Your breakfast should only be one boiled potato (with salt only).

For Lunch and dinner, you will have a vegetable salad with raw vegetables, salt and lemon.

Ingredients

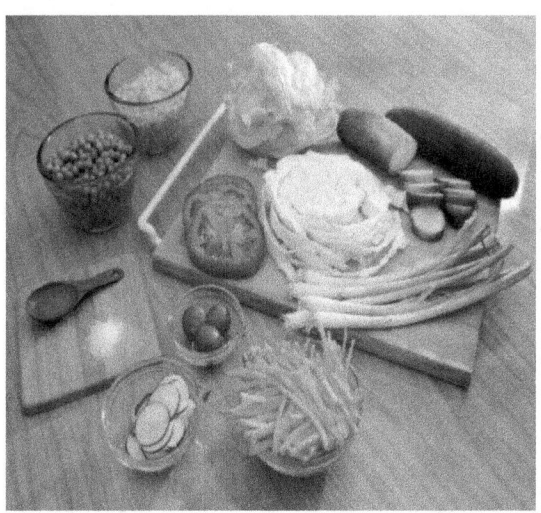

- 10 lettuce leaves

- 1 cabbage, chopped or shredded

- 5 green onions, chopped

- 3 carrots, peeled and sliced into thin strips

- 3 tomatoes, sliced into rings

- 3 tablespoons, fresh lemon juice
- 2 large cucumbers, with skin, sliced
- 3 cherry tomatoes
- 1/2 cup peas
- 1/2 cup corn, boiled
- salt
- celery and broccoli, (optional)
- 1 radish, (optional)

Vegetable Salad Instructions

1. Mix all vegetables in a bowl.
2. Add salt and lemon juice.
3. Refrigerate for one hour. Makes three servings.

Day 3: Fruits and Vegetables

For breakfast, start with fruits, preferably raw and with low sugar. You can drink coffee or green tea for better results.

For lunch and dinner, eat fruits and vegetable salad. Make three servings.

Ingredients for Vegetable Salad

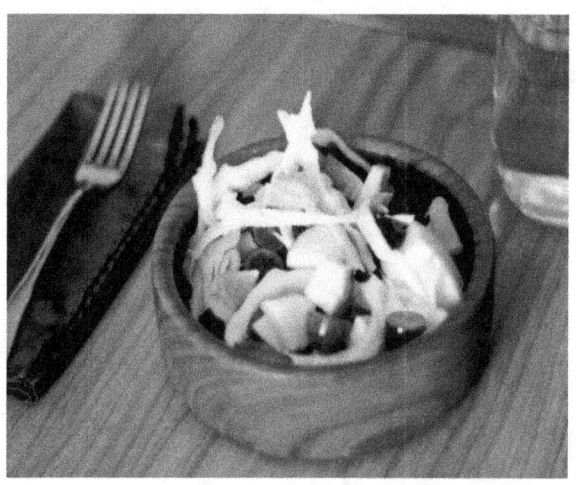

- 3 oranges, peeled and cut into small pieces
- 1 cup green, purple, or red grape halves
- 1/4 cup currants
- 2 apricots or guavas, chopped with seeds removed
- 1 mango, peeled and cubed
- 1/4 grapefruit

- 2 tablespoons fresh lemon juice
- 2 red apples, diced
- 3 cups green cabbage, chopped or shredded

Day 4: Banana's Best

Focus on plain skimmed cow's milk, bananas and homemade soup for Breakfast Lunch and Dinner. In between, you can eat five bananas for a total of eight bananas for this day.

Gunnars (2017) in her article in Authority Nutrition states that studies prove the fact that adding water to your food, and making it into a soup can make you feel more satiated and will cause you to eat significantly fewer calories.

Ingredients for Diet Soup

- 23 ounces water
- 1 onion, cut into rings
- 2 green chilis
- 3 tomatoes
- 1 cabbage
- 2 lettuce leaves
- 1 carrot

Feel free to add salt and lemon juice for a more enriching taste.

Nutrition Facts	
Serving size: 1	
Calories	71
Calories from Fat	0
% Daily Value *	
Fat 0 g	
Carbohydrates 16 g	5%
Fiber 5 g	20%
Protein 3 g	6%
Cholesterol 0 mg	
* The Percent Daily Values are based on a 2,000-calorie diet, so your values may change depending on your calorie needs. The values here may not be 100% accurate because the recipes have not been professionally evaluated nor have they been evaluated by the U.S. FDA.	

Day 5: Tomato Mania

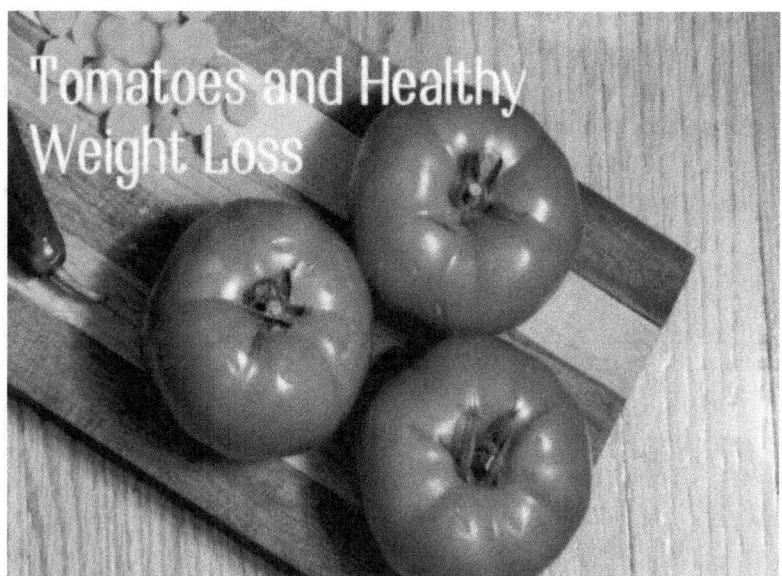

Combining fruits, vegetables and rice to experience full chemical breakdown and weight loss.

Tomatoes are essential for this day, so you need to eat at least six of it. Choose six medium-sized tomatoes and you can add salt and pepper to taste. You can also drink green tea, the weight-loss drink recipe and coffee to go with this diet.

According to Macher (2017), tomatoes are good for weight loss because they are low in fat and carbohydrates. They are fiber-rich and helps you satiate the cravings that keep you from overeating. Apart from these, tomatoes are also low on the glycemic index which means that they do not have a significant effect on your blood sugar levels. It is an amazing weight loss diet because it helps you stat hydrated due to its water content. It is also filled with carotene, vitamin E, A, K, B, iron, magnesium, and phosphorous.

Breakfast	Lunch	Dinner
One grapefruit.	One small bowl of boiled rice.	One bowl soup from Day Four recipe.
One apple.	One bowl of salad from Day Two or Day Three.	One apple.
One orange.	1/2 glass skimmed milk.	Two tomatoes.
Two tomatoes.	Two tomatoes.	

Day 6: Rice, Vegetable, and Soup

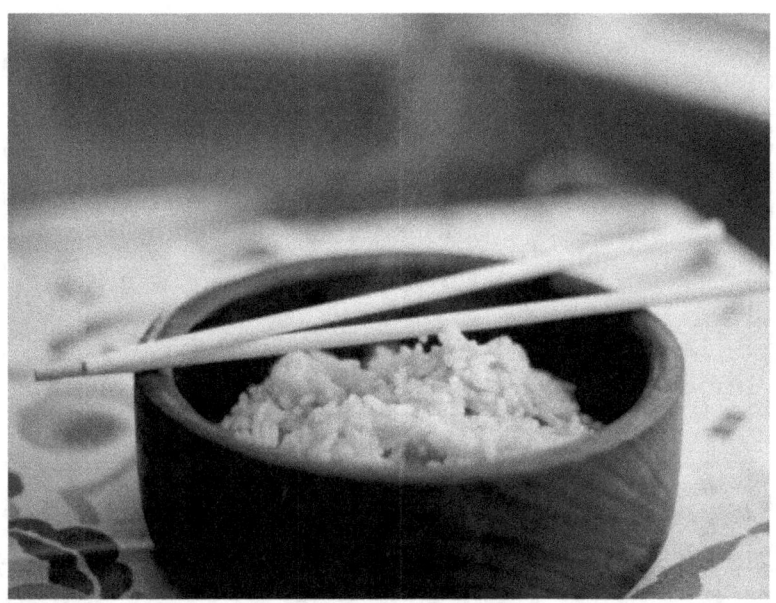

Remember to avoid oil, butter or cheese. You can add lemon juice, salt and pepper for a more enhanced flavor. For breakfast, focus on raw vegetables and one cup of boiled rice, preferable brown for a more nutritious and fuller experience. For lunch and dinner, consider eating one bowl of soup or salad. You can refer to the previous recipes for soup and vegetable salad.

Day 7: Rice, Soup and Juice Diet

Breakfast	Lunch	Dinner
Fresh orange and/or grapefruit juice.	Boiled rice (one bowl).	Diet soup (one bowl).
One apple and one grapefruit.	Raw vegetables (your choice).	Vegetable salad.

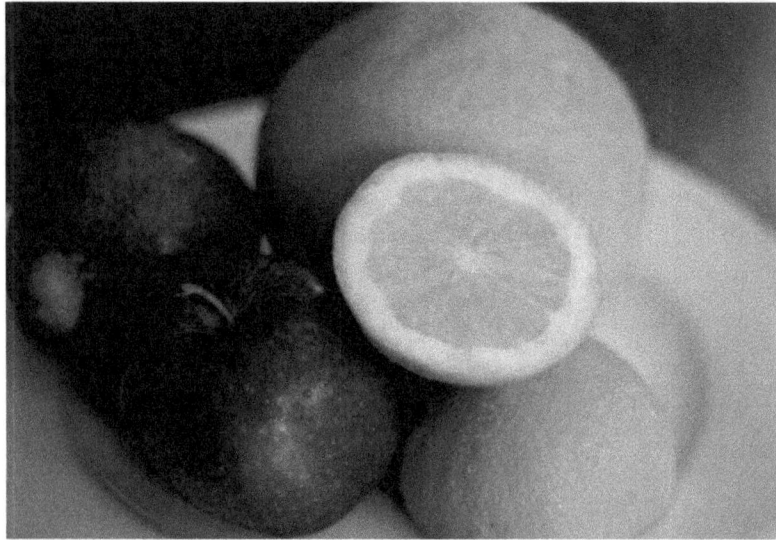

For your juice intake, the quantity is up to you as long as you drink fresh juice. The best fresh juice choice are grapefruit and orange. And the best time to drink it is one hour before and after meals. The best fruits for this diet are strawberries, bananas, apples, oranges, berries and plums. And add vegetables such as onions, carrots and cucumber.

After seven days, measure your weight once again and see instant results. You can keep going on through this process until you reach your desired weight. But you have to remember that reaching your goal takes courage, initiative, cunning, determination and dedication. Without these characteristics, it will be harder for you to stick to your diet plan. This seven-day plan is a very effective means to lose weight given you put yourself on the right mindset and discipline. But with hard work, I know you can do it!

Top 7 Life Hacks in Losing Weight Without Exercise

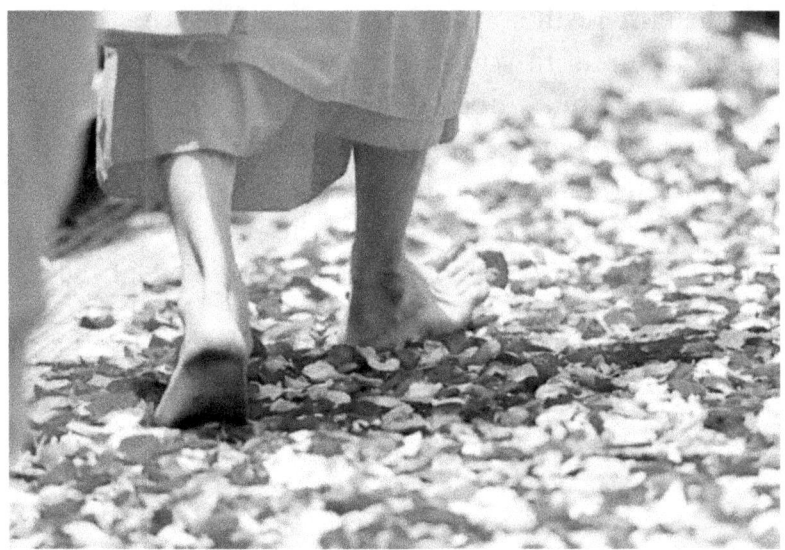

Everyone has the power to change their lives in just simple ways. And in those simple methods come life hacks that can help you in your journey of losing weight. These are practical activities and approaches that you can do to help your body adjust into a leaner, healthier and a slimmer body. According to Maria (2017) Health Reloaded, there are many different life hacks that people can do to lose weight without sweat and exercise.

1. Go for a walk when stressed. Going for long walks is one of the best ways to alleviate tension, pressure and stress which is detrimental to one's diet. As discussed before, stress increases the amount of cortisol in the

body which will intensify your cravings. Taking long walks is a way to alleviate the stress at the same time burn your fat with your diet.

2. Improve your posture. This is one way to stretch the muscles without exercise. This will also help you gain a good shape for your body as you lose weight.

3. Play games. You can play games from Kinect or other arcade games to have fun. This will help you loosen up your muscles and fats so it will be easier for water and other detoxifying foods and beverages to flush them.

4. Go forth on an adventure! You can add different activities in your itinerary such as swimming, snorkeling, wall climbing, and aqua dancing. These will not be a form of exercise for you but a form of adventure, fun, learning, and stress-relief. All of which are essential to weight loss.

5. Volunteering is also one good way to lose weight. This will help you feel occupied, so you can burn the extra calories you take from your diet.

6. If you think you're bored and got nothing to do, you can clean the house, wash the dishes, fix things around, do maintenance work around the house or wash your clothes. In this way, you do not have to sit on the couch all day doing nothing. At least you will become more

productive as you burn your fats towards weight loss.

7. You can also try getting a dog to give you motivation to move around and play with someone. Knowing that dogs have needs, you will have the proper intention to walk around the park and stretch for even a small amount of time. This will help you relieve your stress, and be more efficient on your weight loss diet plan.

Conclusion

Exercise is still a vital part of the human body because it helps strengthen the immune system and build muscles and bones. We also cannot deny that exercise plays a great role in losing weight. However, not all of us has the luxury of time to do so. This is the reason why there are tips and diet plans created to teach people how to lose weight without exercise.

Losing weight without exercise does not necessarily mean that you will become a couch potato for the rest of your diet plan, or better yet, your life. Weight loss is a lot harder than you think. You have to figure out a way to loosen up the fats and calories so your diet can work. And it will not work much if you do not spend your energy once in a while. These life hacks are very efficient even when it seems ridiculous to other people. Before you talk yourself out, why don't you give it a try. There's no harm in trying. You already have the information you need to lose weight despite your busy schedule. It is now up to you to decide if you are willing to be committed to the challenge and process od losing weight without exercise.

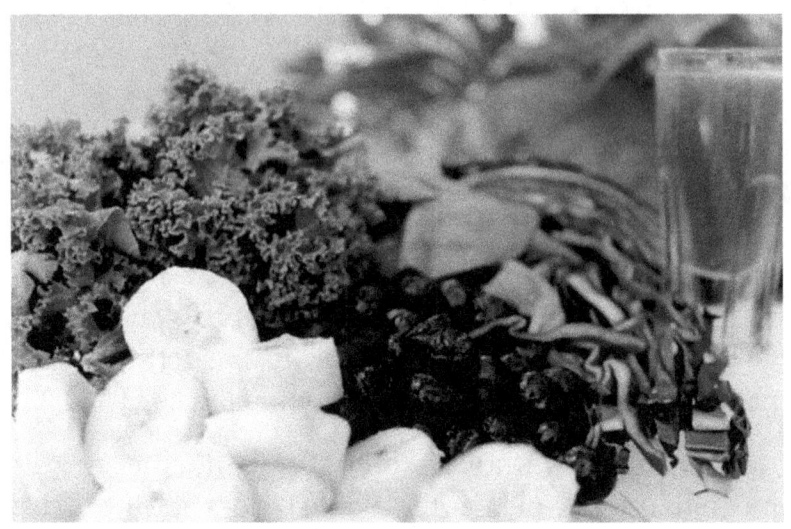

In this book, I have presented various Green smoothie recipes, and the seven-day diet plan to help you change and adjust your food intake on the road to weight loss. I have also included various essential foods which are very effective ways to maintain a healthy body and prevent sickness. If you do not believe that this process can provide the optimum weight goal for you, then you should trust that it can increase your vitality and health as a human being. All of the ingredients mentioned are very effective weight loss diets given they are consumed responsibly.

Losing weight does not happen overnight. It needs persistence, determination, control, and discipline. It is impossible to say that weight loss is as easy as counting, for weight loss takes time and utmost effort. I am sure that all of you have your own reasons for losing weight. But if you have a proper motivation, and determination to do so, I believe that you will be able to lose weight without exercise. When you feel like giving up or quitting, always remember why you started in the first place. Have your vision straight and true. Soon you will be able to wear your skinny jeans and bikini. Soon enough, you will be able to gain more friends and have other people notice and appreciate you. Bullying will no longer an issue and they will no longer call you names. Losing weight has its own perks. Use it to your advantage and finally achieve the body you deserve. Do it for yourself. Change your mind and attitude, and finally change your body.

www.ingramcontent.com/pod-product-compliance
Lightning Source LLC
Chambersburg PA
CBHW072018290526
45787CB00013B/1298